Overcoming:
How I Stopped Living With Anxiety and Depression
Workbook

Randi Coley

ISBN-13: 978-1-959060-05-5

This book is not intended as a substitute for the medical advice of physicians. The reader should regularly consult a physician in matters relating to his/her health, particularly regarding any symptoms that may require diagnosis or medical attention.

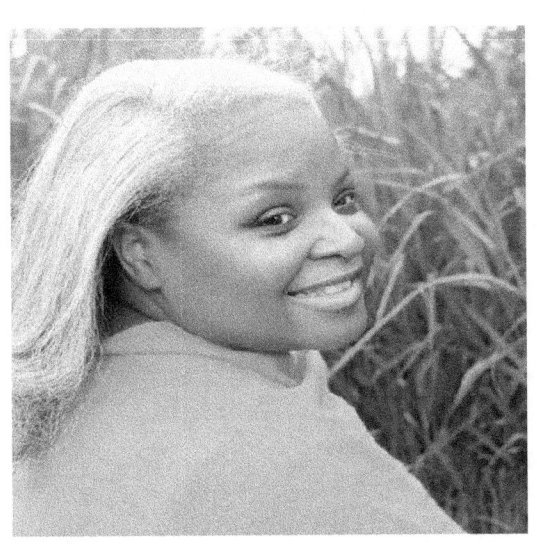

RANDI COLEY

Refined Community Outreach

I am Randi Coley. I believe in my community and the people I serve.

www.randicoley.com

5

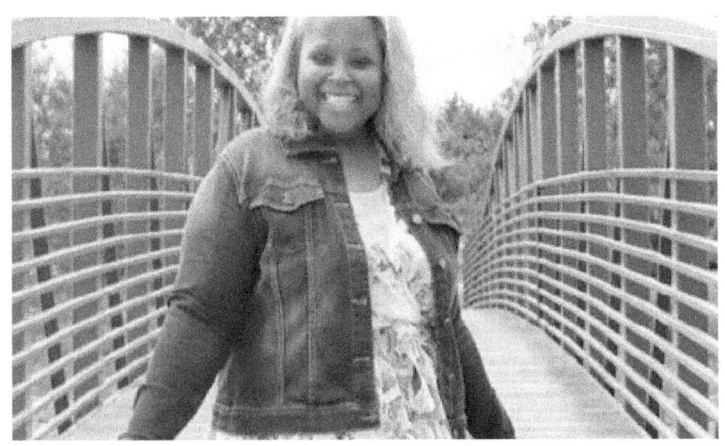

ABOUT RANDI

WELCOME

Randi Coley is an experienced addiction and mental health counselor with a passion for helping individuals overcome their challenges and achieve personal growth. Born in the late 1960s, Randi brings a wealth of knowledge and expertise to her counseling practice.

Randi's educational background includes a bachelor's degree in psychology, which laid the foundation for her deep understanding of human behavior and thought processes. She furthered her studies by obtaining a Master of Health Science in Addictions Studies, specializing in addressing substance abuse issues and related mental health concerns.

COURSE WORKBOOK

```
WHAT  EXPECT

Randi Coley

Complete coaching

Complete counseling
```

```
COURSE WORKBOOK

The road to quieting anxiety and depression through
consistent daily practice to clear the mind.
```

Randi's counseling approach is holistic, incorporating a range of techniques and strategies tailored to each client's unique needs. She believes in the power of mentoring, leadership, and behavioral modification practices to bring about positive change. Through her warm and empathetic demeanor, Randi creates a safe and non-judgmental space where individuals can e

ONLINE COURSE COMMUNICATION

randicoley@hotmail.com
708.581.8448

—

Our business has been set to ensure consistency within our brand, helping to create strong, recognizable, and innovative communications.

—

BUSINESS

Here for consultation, educational, and self-help group experiences.

RESPONSE TIME

Our business has been set to return calls, emails, and correspondence in 24-48 hours.

ONLINE COURSE

THE PROCESS

STEP ONE

Healing the emotional and mental self to address Anxiety and Depression

STEP TWO

Addressing the physical areas that can help soothe and lessen symptoms

STEP THREE

Prayer, Meditation and Spiritual Principles to help lessen anxiety and depression

Introduction

In 1986, while carrying my first child, I became depressed. It was so severe that I suffered from suicidal ideations. Reflecting, I realize that I have had anxiety and depression since being molested as a small child. I had nervous ticks, my hands and knees shook, I bit my fingernails, and couldn't sleep more than a few hours at a time. In 1990, after the birth of my second child, depression and anxiety intensified. After a violent attack in 1993, it progressed to Clinical Depression.

Anxiety and depression are both clinical terms for behaviors that stem from experiences. This is a self-help guide to overcoming anxiety and depression. I did this through everyday practices with deliberate minor changes every day. As a licensed professional, I have employed psychological expertise with everyday practices to lessen the symptoms.

Examples of this are: opening curtains, taking a shower, cutting off phones, taking a 10-minute walk, and journaling. You can overcome anxiety and depression with action, consistency, and patience.

This is not a book suggesting medicine does not work. This is not a book talking against medication. I have used all my tips, while also taking medication. It is a daily struggle to live life with the symptoms of anxiety and depression. Come on this journey with me as I work daily to overcome anxiety and depression.

The below content comes from the DSM 5 and is used for definition only in the content of this work.

Anxiety is defined as "apprehension, uneasiness or nervousness usually over an impending or anticipated illness."

Anxiety Disorder: DSM -5 300.2

Common anxiety signs and symptoms include:

- Feeling nervous, restless, or tense
- Having a sense of impending danger, panic, or doom
- Having an increased heart rate
- Breathing rapidly (hyperventilation)
- Sweating
- Trembling
- Feeling weak or tired
- Trouble concentrating or thinking about anything other than the present worry.
- Having trouble sleeping
- Experiencing gastrointestinal (GI) problems
- Having difficulty controlling worry

- Having the urge to avoid things that trigger anxiety.

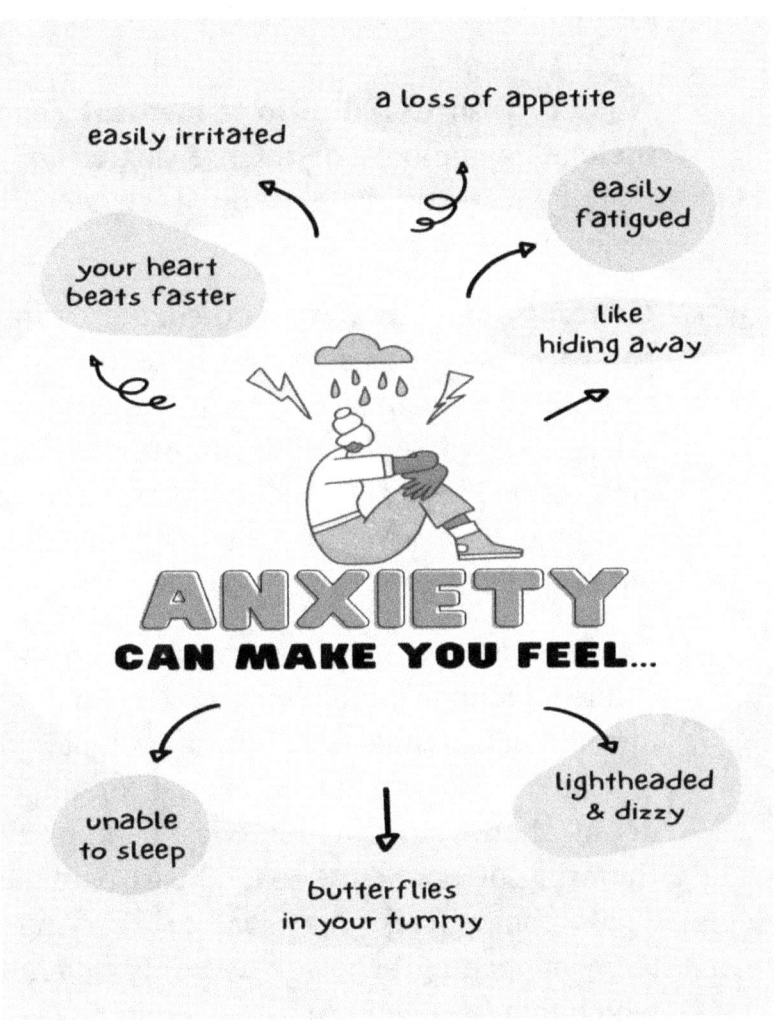

Several types of anxiety disorders exist:

- **Agoraphobia** (ag-uh-ruh-FOE-be-uh) is a type of anxiety disorder in which you fear and often avoid places or situations that might cause you to panic and make you feel trapped, helpless, or embarrassed.

- **Anxiety disorder due to a medical condition** includes symptoms of intense anxiety or panic that are directly caused by a physical health problem.

- **Generalized anxiety disorder** includes persistent and excessive anxiety and worry about activities or events — even ordinary, routine issues. The worry is out of proportion to the actual circumstance, is difficult to control and affects how you feel physically. It often occurs along with other anxiety disorders or depression.

- **Panic disorder** involves repeated episodes of sudden feelings of intense anxiety and fear or terror that reach a peak within minutes (panic attacks). You may have feelings of impending doom, shortness of breath, chest pain, or a rapid, fluttering or pounding heart (heart palpitations). These panic attacks may lead to worrying about them happening again or avoiding situations in which they've occurred.

- **Selective mutism** is a consistent failure of children to speak in certain situations, such as school, even when they can speak in other situations, such as at home with close family members. This can interfere with school, work, and social functioning.

- **Separation anxiety disorder** is a childhood disorder characterized by anxiety that's excessive for the child's developmental level and related to separation from parents or others who have parental roles.

- **Social anxiety disorder (social phobia)** involves high levels of anxiety, fear, and avoidance of social situations due to feelings of embarrassment, self-consciousness, and concern about being judged or viewed negatively by others.

- **Specific phobias** are characterized by major anxiety when you're exposed to a specific object or situation and a desire to avoid it. Phobias provoke panic attacks in some people.

- **Substance-induced anxiety disorder** is characterized by symptoms of intense anxiety or panic that are a direct result of misusing drugs, taking medications, being exposed to a toxic substance, or withdrawal from drugs.

- Other specified anxiety disorders and unspecified anxiety disorders are terms for anxiety or phobias that don't meet the exact criteria for any other anxiety disorders but are significant enough to be distressing and disruptive.

When to see a doctor

See your doctor if:

- You feel like you're worrying too much, and it's interfering with your work, relationships, or other parts of your life.

- Your fear, worry, or anxiety is upsetting to you and difficult to control.

- You feel depressed, have trouble with alcohol or drug use, or have other mental health concerns along with anxiety.

- You think your anxiety could be linked to a physical health problem.

- You have suicidal thoughts or behaviors — if this is the case, seek emergency treatment immediately.

Your worries may not go away on their own, and they may get worse over time if you don't seek help. See your doctor or a mental health provider before your anxiety gets worse. It's easier to treat if you get help early.

Causes

The causes of anxiety disorders aren't fully understood. Life experiences such as traumatic events appear to trigger anxiety disorders in people who are already prone to anxiety. Inherited traits also can be a factor.

Medical causes

For some people, anxiety may be linked to an underlying health issue. In some cases, anxiety signs and symptoms are the first indicators of a medical illness. If your doctor suspects your anxiety may have a medical cause, he or she may order tests to look for signs of a problem.

Examples of medical problems that can be linked to anxiety include:

- Heart disease

- Diabetes

- Thyroid problems, such as hyperthyroidism

- Respiratory disorders, such as chronic obstructive pulmonary disease (COPD) and asthma

- Drug misuse or withdrawal.

- Withdrawal from alcohol, anti-anxiety medications (benzodiazepines) or other medications

- Chronic pain or irritable bowel syndrome

- Rare tumors that produce certain fight-or-flight hormones

Sometimes anxiety can be a side effect of certain medications.

It's possible that your anxiety may be due to an underlying medical condition if:

- You don't have any blood relatives (such as a parent or sibling) with an anxiety disorder.

- You didn't have an anxiety disorder as a child.

- You don't avoid certain things or situations because of anxiety.

- You have a sudden occurrence of anxiety that seems unrelated to life events, and you didn't have a previous history of anxiety.

Risk factors.

These factors may increase your risk of developing an anxiety disorder:

- **Trauma.** Children who endured abuse or trauma or witnessed traumatic events are at higher risk of developing an anxiety disorder at some point in life. Adults who experience a traumatic event can also develop anxiety disorders.

- **Stress due to an illness.** Having a health condition or serious illness can cause significant worry about issues such as your treatment and your future.

- **Stress buildup.** A big event or a buildup of smaller stressful life situations may trigger excessive anxiety — for example, a death in the family, work stress, or ongoing worry about finances.

- **Personality.** People with certain personality types are more prone to anxiety disorders than others are.

- **Other mental health disorders.** People with other mental health disorders, such as depression, often also have an anxiety disorder.

- **Having blood relatives with an anxiety disorder.** Anxiety disorders can run in families.

- **Drugs or alcohol.** Drug or alcohol use or misuse or withdrawal can cause or worsen anxiety.

Complications

Having an anxiety disorder does more than make you worry. It can also lead to, or worsen, other mental and physical conditions, such as:

- Depression (which often occurs with an anxiety disorder) or other mental health disorders.

- Substance misuse

- Trouble sleeping (insomnia)

- Digestive or bowel problems

- Headaches and chronic pain

- Social isolation

- Problems functioning at school or work.

- Poor quality of life

- Suicide

Prevention

There's no way to predict for certain what will cause someone to develop an anxiety disorder, but you can take steps to reduce the impact of symptoms if you're anxious:

- **Get help early.** Anxiety, like many other mental health conditions, can be harder to treat if you wait.

- **Stay active.** Participate in activities that you enjoy and that make you feel good about yourself. Enjoy social interaction and caring relationships, which can lessen your worries.

- **Avoid alcohol or drug use.** Alcohol and drug use can cause or worsen anxiety. If you're addicted to any of these substances, quitting can make you anxious. If you can't quit on your own, see your doctor or find a support group to help you.

"Be careful for nothing; but in every thing by prayer and supplication with thanksgiving let your requests be made known unto God. "
—Philippians 4:6
" Do not be anxious about anything, but in every situation, by prayer and petition, with thanksgiving, present your requests to God. "
—Philippians 4:6 NIV

My real healing came from a combination of several techniques. Some people don't believe in God, I do. The very first part of my healing came by way of repentance, prayer and studying the Bible. I believe healing starts with an acknowledgment of what belongs to you and what part you have no control over. The second part of healing, I know some church folks are going to say it is not necessary, but I also sought counseling and medical(medication) intervention. The third part is the use of daily practices that help to lessen symptoms of anxiety and depression.

To keep anxiety and depression symptoms lessened, I keep a routine necessary to help my daily functioning.

Step One

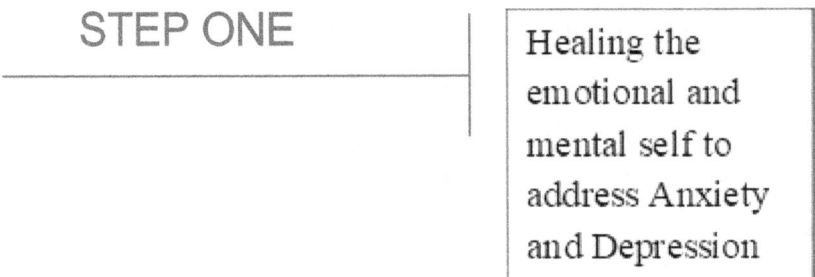

STEP ONE | Healing the emotional and mental self to address Anxiety and Depression

Starting this process was very difficult due to dealing with step one. Addressing childhood trauma. In many instances, this was a process that was painful and overwhelming. I had to face the pain of my past. I was the youngest child of seven. I am also a twin. I was a twin that had an opposite. I was dark, and she was light. I was short, and she was tall. She was slender, and I was stocky and thick.

As I began to work on this workbook, I had to face myself. I also had to face my own trauma. In doing so, I am going to be very transparent. I most likely had, at the beginning of this process, the mental age of a five-year-old. I was molested between the ages of three and five years of age. I also dealt with colorism, favoritism, and other abuses within my family. There were several attempts at healing over the years, and to be perfectly clear, I am still dealing with the side effects of maladaptive behaviors I tried to use as a method to heal from childhood trauma. I was an extremely shy child who was so introverted that I shut down in new situations. I was so introverted that when I was in first grade because my sister was not near me and we were not in the same class, I refused to do any work, talk, or engage in the class. Because of this, I was left back in the first grade. This was the catalyst for a lot of stress and terrible treatment I experienced over the next several years by all kinds of people in my life. All of which caused a lot of emotional traumas.

In the easiest sense, I addressed my inner child as part of my emotional healing. By embracing her mentally first. And by encouraging her and building my self-esteem. I also know that it is a daily practice that works in helping to maintain my mental health. Part of my emotional healing starts with forgiving myself. And writing a letter to the little girl inside.

A Letter to my Younger Self, the Child that Lives

Little girl, little girl… remember you are always a twin.

You are an individual, sharp, beautiful and intelligent.

Keep your own personality, know you are beautiful when others look superficially.

Looks matter to some when others value intellect and integrity.

You value to some, will be your personality. You must value yourself to maintain your dignity.

Hold on to your "no" don't let it go.

When the "boys" come, it's not you it's their "issues" that gaslight, manipulate and victimize.

It's the lies, you've been fed your entire life.

You are more than enough. Live in peace.

* I have noticed that when I am around certain people, they cause me to be anxious. Certain situations cause me anxiety. Code switching can cause me to have anxious feelings. I also have learned that when people treat me as if I am incompetent, it can cause me to have anxious feelings*

Another way I deal with my childhood trauma is to write in a journal/notebook. I assess my mental and emotional health daily. Doing this helps me to deal with everyday reminders or mental stressors that bother me daily. Yes, life is bothersome when you have anxiety. Anything can trigger the symptoms of anxiety. However, once you learn what causes your anxiety to activate you can control the severity and the way you cope. I check my mood. I have a list of things to complete and some changes to make. I write about daily success and what worked to ease my anxiety symptoms.

The following page is a mental assessment to use as a gauge for a self-assessment to use daily.

Self Assessement

Productivity

- [ ]
- [ ]
- [ ]
- [ ]
- [ ]
- [ ]
- [ ]
- [ ]
- [ ]
- [ ]
- [ ]

Life Assessement

- [ ]
- [ ]
- [ ]
- [ ]
- [ ]
- [ ]
- [ ]
- [ ]
- [ ]
- [ ]

I overcame anxiety today list

Something that eased anxiety today.

REVIEW

_____

_____

_____

_____

_____

_____

_____

_____

_____

_____

_____

Step Two

Addressing the physical areas that can help soothe and lessen symptoms.

STEP TWO

My real healing came from a combination of several techniques. Some people don't believe in God, I do. The very first part of my healing came by way of repentance, prayer, and studying the Bible. I believe healing starts with an acknowledgment of what belongs to you and what part you have no control over. The second part of healing, I know some church folks are going to say it is not necessary, but I also sought counseling and medical(medication) intervention. The third part is the use of daily practices that help to lessen symptoms of anxiety and depression. To keep anxiety and depression symptoms lessened, I keep a routine necessary to help my daily functioning.

1. When I wake up each morning, because depression and anxiety can lead to poor hygiene habits, I use a routine. When I get up to go to the restroom first thing in the morning, I take everything for my shower with me. I start the

shower, while I use the facilities. When I finish, I take my shower. (so even if I go lay back down, I have already taken my shower).

2. The next thing I do is open all my blinds and curtains in the morning before I move around. To let in natural light. Which helps mood.

3. Because of anxiety I tend to have nervous energy or "fidgeting". Like biting fingernails, leg rocking or cracking knuckles. One of the ways I combat this is by keeping my hands busy. I type, use a squeeze ball, chew gum (instead of eating). Or I exercise.

4. When I have a panic attack in situations where anxiety comes on fast, I use deep slow breathing while closing my eyes. I also talk to myself to calm down. (Girl, you got this. No one is as strong as you, you will be okay. Know it.)

5. Another way I overcome my anxiety diagnosis is to combat physical symptoms by regular exercise or doing something I enjoy. Before Covid 19, I walked 4 miles a day, during the covid shutdowns. I started to write daily as a coping mechanism. I started working on crafts again and sewing. These are things I enjoy that help protect my sanity.

These are the general ways I used to overcome anxiety

every day. These ways have worked for some of my physical behaviors from anxiety. All these behaviors are the positive ones that have survived after years of personal growth.

In an effort to be transparent… when I initially started the process of healing, I did not learn appropriate coping skills. Originally, I had maladaptive behaviors that could cause not only health problems   but also could cause death. Previous behaviors like, smoking, sex addiction, eating disorders, self-isolation due to anxiety, sleeping too much due to depression, and lashing out at others when overwhelmed or angry, lying, and low self-esteem.

A QUICK NOTE TO YOU…

I KNOW THAT YOU WILL BE ANXIOUS DUE TO INTERNAL RESPONSES SO PLEASE:

To protect your peace ....

It's okay to cancel a commitment.

It's okay to not take the call.

It's okay to change your mind.

It's okay to take a day off.

It's okay to speak up.

It's okay to be alone.

It's okay to let go.

It's okay to say no

REVIEW

_____

_____

_____

_____

_____

_____

_____

_____

_____

_____

Step Three

STEP THREE

| Prayer, Meditation and Spiritual Principles to help lessen anxiety and depression. |

As part of my healing came by way of repentance, prayer, and studying the Bible. I believe healing starts with an acknowledgment of what belongs to you and what part you have no control over.

In 1996, when I dedicated my life to GOD, I was already fully ingrained in maladaptive behaviors like drinking alcohol, casual (addictive)sexual activity, and smoking cigarettes (a pack a day.) I had a newborn and was soon to be seven years old. I was living on my own for the first time in a while with no money, man, or enough education to support myself.

The thought of that sent my depression and anxiety over the edge. I was already in depression due to the recent break from my then drug addict ex. Post partum depression as well as a very domineering mother that pointed out how bleak my life looked.

Previously, I struggled with self-confidence, and for

this reason I did not finish anything in my life timely. I struggled with how to make decisions that were sound in judgement, less impulsively, and face the consequences if my life as the single mother of not just one child but two. It was when the symptoms started after a few years of out-of-control stuff that I knew I needed help.

The first thing I used when I dedicated my life to GOD was prayer.

I follow a routine every morning of praying when I wake up, usually between three and four a.m.

I must admit I struggle with listening, so for many years, it was hard for me to sit still and allow God to speak to me. It wasn't until 2006 when I had a trial of my faith, that I learned how to listen to God's voice and guidance.

The scripture that I learned I reference to this is at the start of first step.

" Be careful for nothing; but in every thing by prayer and supplication with thanksgiving let your requests be made known unto God."
—Philippians 4:6

This took me into a study of the word anxious. Which is basically an extreme fear or worry. When a person worries, they are stealing the opportunity to have peace and joy.

The next scripture I came upon as I studied peace was in Psalms.

Ps. 30:4-5(KJV). Sing unto the Lord, O ye saints and his, and give thanks at the remembrance of his holiness. For his anger endureth but for the moment, in his favor is life. Weeping may endure for a night, but joy cometh in the morning.

At times in life, we are so inundated with the cares of every day. In that we forget to be grateful for the simple things in life, like food, shelter, and clothes on our backs. A friend of mine laughed one day. And, in her laughter, she told me to laugh with me. She literally took me in her arms and tickled and shook me until I laughed out loud. Then asked me to list 5 things that I was grateful for.

So, when I gave her my list, she gave me instructions to list 3 things I am grateful for every day. She then told me that as a believer in GOD or a woman of faith, it is my responsibility to be grateful in my life.

"1Thess.5:18- In everything give thanks: for this is the will of God in Christ Jesus concerning you."

What I learned was to find a way of being grateful and voicing it. "In the church many times people are told, let everything that have breathe praises ye the Lord." So, I began by starting the day with gratitude. I say three things I am grateful for when I wake up before I touch the floor. When I pray, the first words of prayer start with …Thank you, Lord.

After a few weeks, I noticed every day with gratitude and giving thanks. I felt lighter.

I walked four miles a day. I changed my diet and was meeting with my therapist weekly. I also would like to add I was taking the prescribed anti-anxiety medication.

There was a time when I was able to be weaned off medication with the help of counseling, prayer, and my therapist. Also, life was not stressful, and I was very strict in my routine. All of this helped me to get better.

In recent years – since 2016, when my daughter was incarcerated and then with quarantine during Covid 19, I had to start taking anti-anxiety and depression medication again. Just meditating on the goodness and blessings in my life has made so much difference.

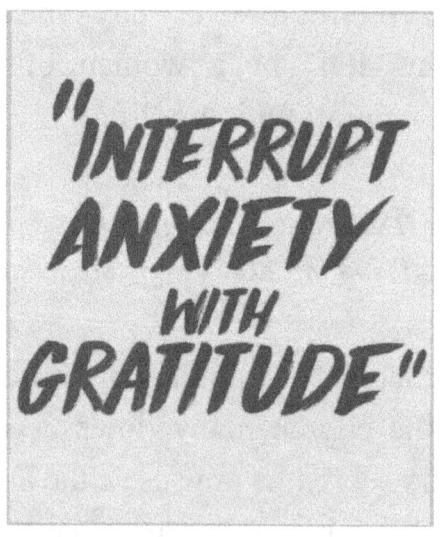

Note from the Author:

I hope this workbook helped you. I have made this very simple. I did that for the benefit of anyone suffering. I know you may feel like it's impossible not to feel anxious. I can tell you that it is.

I will be holding an online class where we dive deeper into healing techniques and your best options.

EndNote

When I started this journey, the intention was to write this after the mini podcast that I have been dropping topics in for over a year. During this time of writing, I became ill. I struggled with self-sabotage and became frustrated. When I reviewed the submission of this project, I realized the original submission was not only incomplete it was mangled with sentences that did not make sense. I used the voice command to write when I was under the weather, and it was a hot mess on paper.

I had to get out of my own way and give myself a moment to allow God to work in his lovingkindness. I am a month past my deadline. I have another project that was born through this process. I let go of something I hoped for to get to this point. The point of this all is to deal with everything I dreamed of. Let each thing go to live in the purpose for which I was intended.

Never give up your purpose for a daydream.

Randi

About Randi Coley

Born the last year of the 60s, Educated with a bachelor's in psychology and a Master of Health Science in Addictions studies. She is an addiction and mental counselor who has worked in the helping and social services field for twenty years. She is an entrepreneur with two community outreach organizations. Her goal through various forms of media is to educate, inspire, motivate, and uplift by words of inspiration, mentoring, leadership, and behavioral modification practices for change.

Coming soon...

GIVING THEM THEIR FLOWERS:
A variety of anecdotal short stories with life lessons and salutes to those who have affected me over the course of my 50-plus years of life. That impact may have been knowledge, taught me a skill, or even gut-checked me. I have written about it and thanked them for this work. Gospel singer James Cleveland sang the song "Give Me My Flowers." I can't sing, so here is my offering.

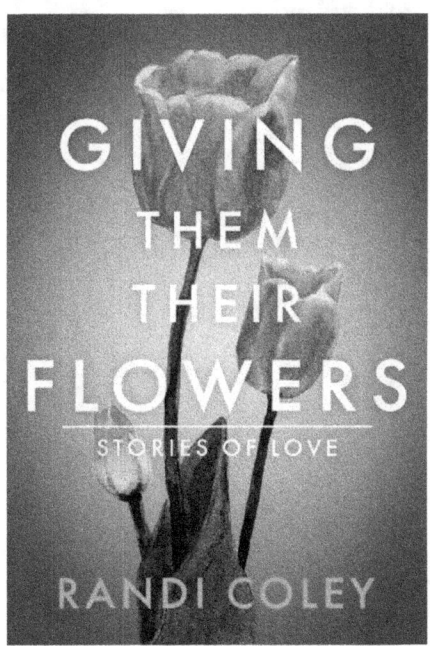

FREEDOM:

The words from the pen of a ready writer. Psalms 45:1. Poetry, Prose, and words of inspiration. A collection of writings. While passing the time, sometimes I just write it down and expound on it later. Writing is where I let my Freedom live.

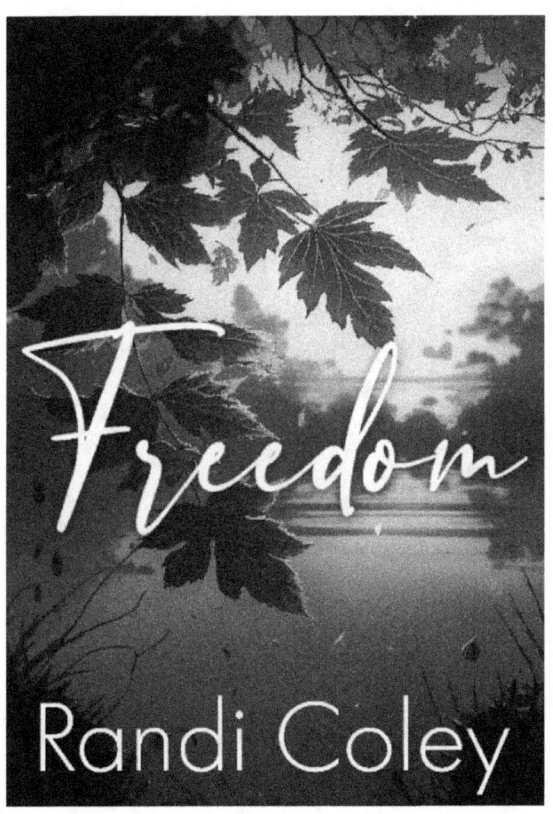

Already Available …

In 2006, after a trial of my faith, God began to deal with my heart and guide me toward his word, his way for me to live and love. It was not the love of a "man" or mankind. It was his eternal Godly love. In the beginning, I called it a "Journey into Love."

As time went on, at the next phase, I called it "Grandmother's Chronicles." At this present time, I call it "Refinement Time." All three of these are different names

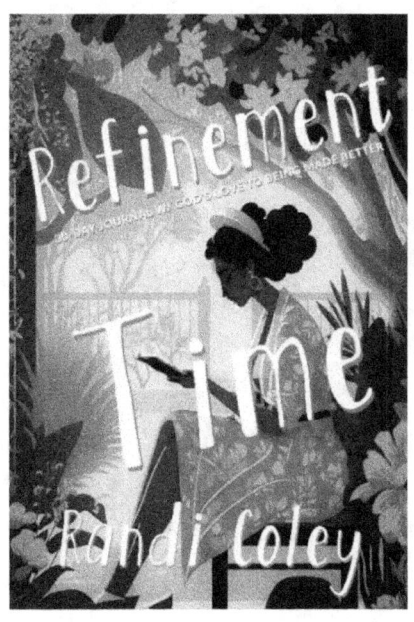

that all take me to and are references for the same thing. The references for being made better. That is, I can be made whole through my life in God: In His love, and through the guidance of His word.

As a licensed counselor, I have added a touch of Psycho-Social tips to apply with scripture and journaling. It's Refinement Time. Let's be made better.

A beautifully crafted 150-page journal for you to write the desires of your heart and watch them manifest.

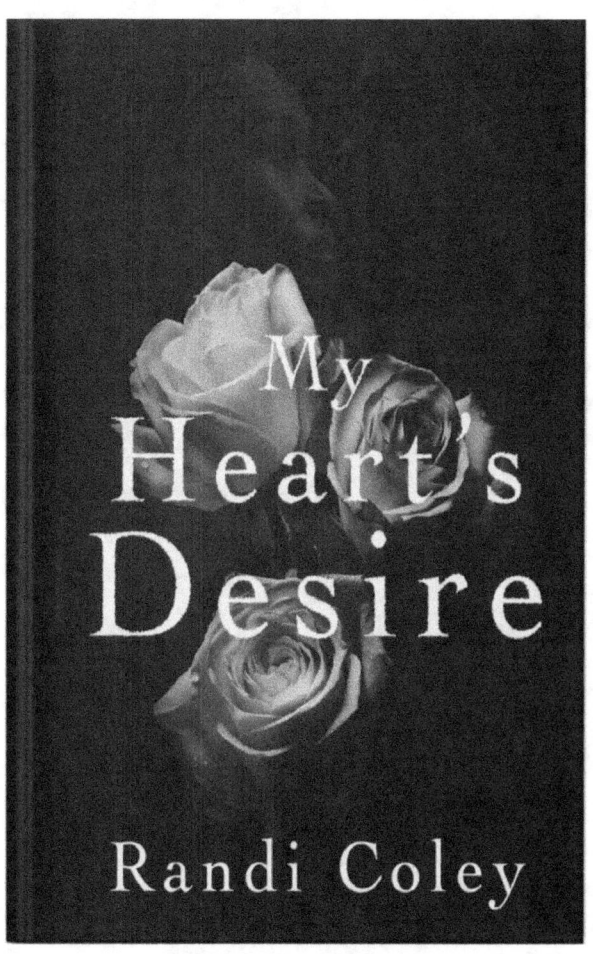